Understanding Aromatherapy

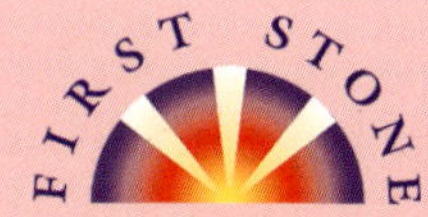

Contents

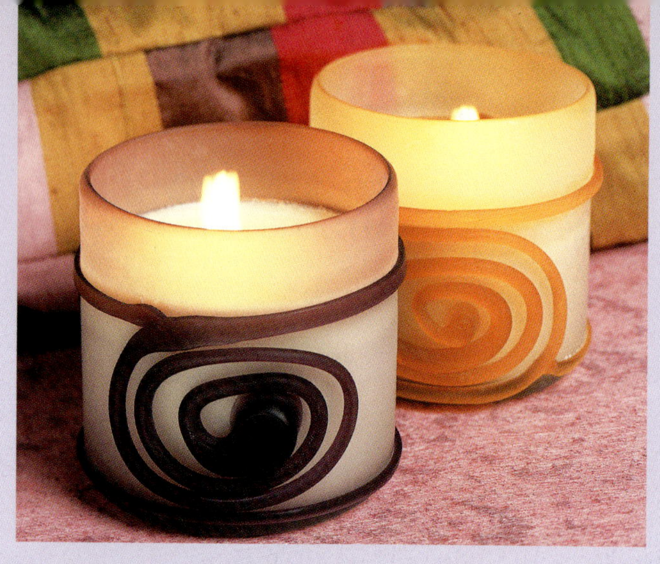

1

Introducing Aromatherapy

Aromatherapy involves the therapeutic use of essential oils that have been extracted from herbs, flowers, fruits and trees.

ESSENTIAL OILS

As well as giving plants their distinctive 'aromas', essential oils contain complex chemical compounds that have a range of physiological and psychological effects. The aroma of an essential oil may inspire a range of responses, and may also contribute to the sense of well-being associated with receiving aromatherapy, but it is the chemical constituents that give an oil its specific healing properties.

Strictly speaking, the term 'aromatherapy' means the use of fragrances to treat and prevent health problems solely by means of inhalation. However, essential oils can also be absorbed through the skin, and, in practice, essential oils may be used in massage, baths, and direct application to the skin. Occasionally, oils may be given orally – but only by qualified aromatherapists.

ORIGINS

No one person can really be credited with the 'invention' of aromatherapy, as the use of essential oils goes back to ancient times. However, a French chemist called René-Maurice Gattefossé was the first to use the term.

While working in his family's perfume factory, Gattefossé burnt his hand. To relieve the pain he plunged it into a nearby container of neat lavender oil. Much to his surprise, his burns healed within hours and without scarring.

Gattefossé went on to investigate the properties of other oils, eventually publishing his findings in a book called *Aromathérapie* in 1937. Other researchers around the world were also exploring the properties of essential oils, although, in many cases, they were often unaware of each other's work.

It was another Frenchman, Dr. Jean Valnet, who was most influential in the development of aromatherapy as it is practised today. During the Second World War, he used essential oils as antiseptics in the treatment of war wounds. Over the next 20 years, he continued to use and explore their properties. His major work, which was also called *Aromathérapie,* was published in 1964, and it has inspired many to follow his lead.

In the 1950s and 60s, aromatherapist Marguerite Maury reintroduced the idea of using essential oils diluted in vegetable oil in combination with massage. This was a practice that had fallen into disuse for almost 1,000 years.

WHO CAN IT HELP?
Aromatherapy is suitable for everyone. When used properly, it enhances well-being, relieves stress and helps to prevent ill health. It can also be used in the treatment of many illnesses and conditions.

Essential oils can be safely used at home, provided that instructions are followed carefully (see Chapter Six). In this context, most common health problems will respond well to amateur aromatherapy.

When dealing with more

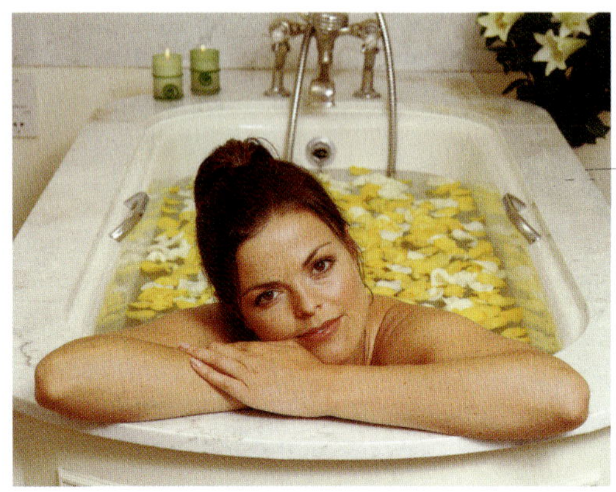

Essential aromatherapy oils can be safely used at home in many cases.

complex or serious conditions, aromatherapy is likely to be of help only when practised by a trained therapist.

As with many complementary therapies, aromatherapy can also be used in conjunction with other natural therapies, and as a complement to conventional medical treatment.

RESEARCH FINDINGS

For such a popular therapy, there is surprisingly little research supporting the therapeutic claims of aromatherapy.

There is evidence that aromas have psychological benefits. Research into the effect that essential oils have on the nervous system found that changes in electrical activity of the brain (stimulation or sedation) often correlates with traditional properties ascribed to particular essential oils. Of course, it may be that these changes are the result of our expectations, rather than any inherent effect of the oil.

However, we know that essential oils can be absorbed into the bloodstream by inhalation and topical application. Research has also shown that essential oils often have antiseptic qualities and a anti-microbial activity. Furthermore, essential oils can enhance the sedative effect of massage, they can act as anti-inflammatories, they can relieve pain, and they also have digestive and sedative properties.

Clinical studies using individual essential oils are limited, but have shown that the following essential oils can help a range of problems:

- Lavender oil will heal burns and cold sores, as well as helping to relieve stress and insomnia.
- Tea tree oil has anti-fungal and anti-bacterial properties. It can effectively treat several skin infections and MRSA (a bug that is resistant to many other treatments).
- Peppermint oil is good for irritable bowel syndrome.
- Thyme oil is good for migraines.

ELEMENT OF TRUST

Aromatherapy, like so many other complementary therapies, is founded on a body of knowledge built up over time. Aromatherapy practitioners, using essential oils every day of their working lives, have a great deal of experience to draw on. Few people have had the time, money or the inclination to clinically test what they believe to work.

Although a therapist may not be able to prove that a particular essential oil or combination of oils will help the problem you have brought to them, it does not mean that the treatment will not work. It simply means that you have to take it on trust. For some people this may be unacceptable, in which case aromatherapy may not be for them. However, for those with an open-minded approach to complementary therapies, aromatherapy may be just what they are looking for.

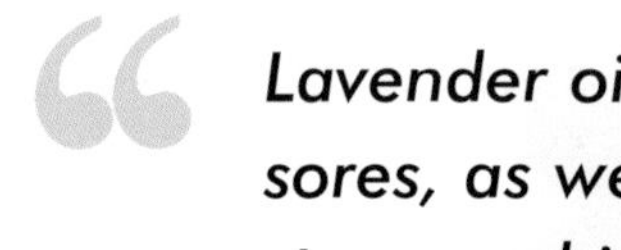

Lavender oil will heal burns and cold sores, as well as helping to relieve stress and insomnia

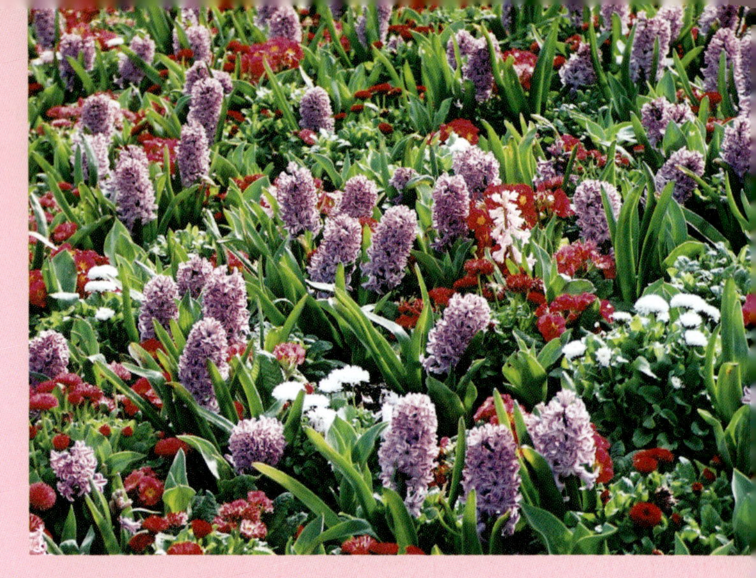

2 A Brief History

Aromatherapy is one of the most ancient therapies, and has been practised for thousands of years.

Archaeological evidence indicates that the people of the Indus Valley (in modern-day Pakistan) were distilling oils 5,000 years ago.

Egyptian papyrus, dating to around 1,550BC and thought to be a compilation of more ancient works, also describes remedies and methods of application not very different from those used in herbal medicine and aromatherapy today. Further east, Chinese and Indian writings dating from 2,000BC describe the use of aromatics for medicinal and religious practices.

The Ancient Greeks added to Egyptian knowledge, using olive oil to absorb plant aromas, for example.

ROMAN AROMAS

When the Romans employed Greek physicians, the use of aromatics spread throughout the Roman Empire. Graeco-Roman texts were, in turn, translated and added to by the Arabs, who went on to develop ways of distilling essential oils.

MEDICINAL VALUE

Herbs and other plants were being used as medicines by the earliest settlers in northern Europe. It is highly probable that the Europeans' knowledge of the healing properties contained in their oils would have been added to with the coming of the Romans in the first century AD.

By the Middle Ages, aromatic oils from the East were arriving in Europe, partly through trade and also with Crusaders returning from their Holy Wars.

The 16th century saw great strides being made in the distillation and use of essential oils, mainly in Germany. Works surviving from that period detail the medicinal value of an increasing number of essential oils. Some of these works were translated into English, but they had little impact in Britain until the following century.

The 17th century was the Golden Age for English

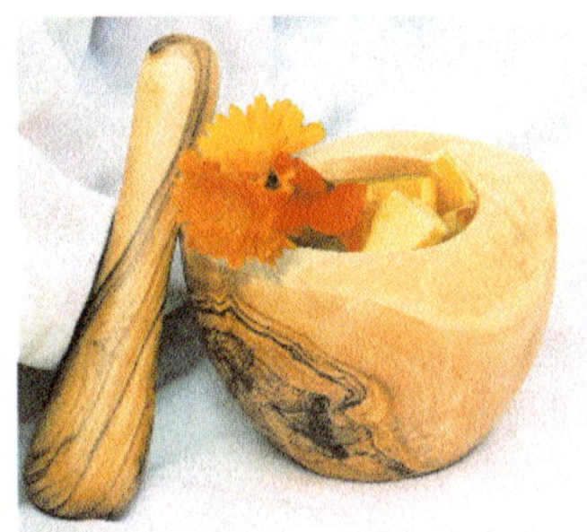

herbalists, including Nicholas Culpeper and John Gerade. Essential oils were much more widely used, both by herbalists and doctors. This was a trend that continued into the 18th century.

During the Renaissance, the distillation process was industrialised, and there was interest in the chemical constituents of the oils. More serious scientific exploration of essential oils began in the 19th century, although, as the century progressed, essential oils were used less and less.

By the 1940s the recognised medical applications of essential oils had largely been reduced to the role of flavouring agents for conventional medicines.

REVIVAL
It took Gattefossé's discoveries and the pioneering work of Dr. Jean Valnet (not to mention valuable contributions by researchers and doctors as far afield as Japan, the former Soviet Union, Italy and America) to rekindle interest in the therapeutic value of essential oils and to bring about the development of modern-day aromatherapy.

MODERN AROMATHERAPY
In the UK, aromatherapy has, in the matter of a few decades, grown from a largely unknown 'beauty treatment' to a therapy practised by a huge number of trained therapists who are members of well-organised regulatory bodies.

Aromatherapy is now widely used by nurses and doctors within the health service. On the high street, aromatherapy kits and individual bottles of oils are on sale in many pharmacies. In bookshops, there are plenty of self-help publications to be found that explain how to use aromatherapy at home.

COMPLEMENTARY THERAPIES
Many commentators credit the Thalidomide tragedy of the 1960s with provoking a crisis of confidence in conventional medicine. (Thalidomide was used to treat morning sickness in pregnant women. However, when the women gave birth, it was discovered that the babies had suffered terrible physical deformities as a result.) Whether this had an effect on people's confidence is difficult to assess. However, it is the case that, in recent years, people have begun to explore alternative ways of tackling health problems. The growth in popularity of complementary therapies – aromatherapy being just one of these – would seem to be part of this movement.

3

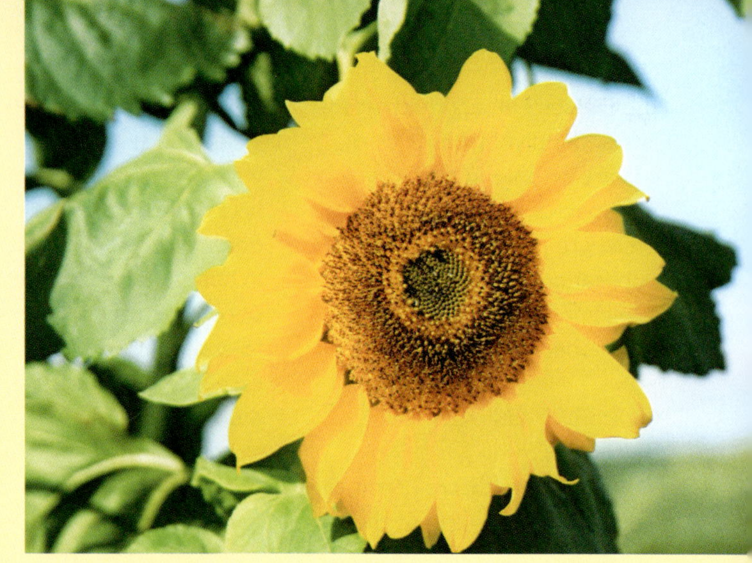

Essential Oils

Essential oils are volatile (able to evaporate) organic constituents of fragrant plants and herbs.

Essential oils can be extracted from flowers, leaves, fruit, seeds, wood, roots, rhizomes, resin and bark. In a plant's lifecycle, the oils are involved in growth and reproduction, attracting pollinating insects, repelling predators, and protecting against disease.

Properties of essential oils include being non-oily, aromatic, volatile, slightly soluble in water (about 20 per cent), inflammable, and able to dissolve in fats (such as vegetable oils) and pure alcohol.

THERAPEUTIC PROPERTIES

Each essential oil is composed of several hundred different chemical constituents, which, taken together, are believed to give the oil its specific therapeutic properties.

The main compounds involved are hydrocarbons called terpenes, and oxygenated compounds, including esters, aldehydes, ketones, alcohols, phenols and oxides. Lactones, sulphur and nitrogen compounds are also found in some oils.

Analysis of these compounds suggests they have particular therapeutic properties. For example, the esters are relaxants and anti-spasmodics (they relieve spasm of the smooth muscle); aldehydes are anti-infectious; and some terpenes have a cortisone-like action. Other compounds have anti-allergic properties.

PURITY

The quality and the exact chemical content of an essential oil is affected by how and where it is grown, and by the way in which it is extracted. For best results, essential oils should be grown organically and extracted without the addition of other chemicals.

In the perfume industry essential oils are usually adulterated with synthetic chemicals. The reason for this is because synthetic chemicals increase productivity and

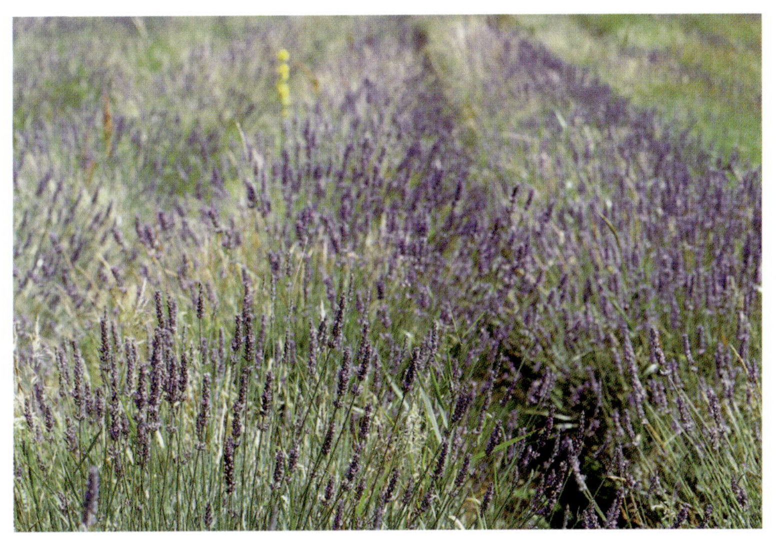

For best results, it is important that essential oils are extracted from organically grown plants, such as this lavender.

stabilise the perfume.
However, these chemicals can
also reduce or remove the
therapeutic effect of the oil, as
well as possibly increasing
toxicity.

EXTRACTION

Most essential oils are
extracted by distillation, but
maceration, expression and
solvent extraction methods
can also be used, depending
on the oil. Distillation involves
placing the plant material in a
still and passing steam under
pressure through it. The heat
causes the tiny sacs containing
essential oil to burst open and
the oil rapidly evaporates.

Steam and essential oil
vapour pass along a pipe,
which is water-cooled. This
condenses the vapours back to
a liquid form. The water and
essential oil are easily
separated because the oil
floats on the top of the water.
High standards of production
are necessary, as incomplete
distillation may reduce the oil's
therapeutic effects.

The yield of essential oil
from this process varies from

plant to plant. On average, 70kg (154lb) of plant material will yield around 1kg (2lb) of essential oil. However, some plants have a much smaller yield. Jasmine oil, for example, requires some eight million jasmine flowers to yield just 1kg (2lb) of oil. Similarly, more than 6,000kg (13,227lb) of rose petals are required to produce 1kg (2lb) of rose oil.

Not surprisingly, jasmine and rose oil are the most expensive essential oils – at around 50 times the cost of most others!

HOW ESSENTIAL OILS WORK

Aromatherapists believe that essential oils enter the body through the olfactory system and the skin. It is thought that, when inhaled, the oils act as a sort of trigger on the central nervous system. When applied to the skin, the oils are believed to permeate through to the blood capillaries and cell tissues.

Only a small amount of essential oil is absorbed through the skin. Over time, most of the molecules of the 'aroma' disperse in the air and

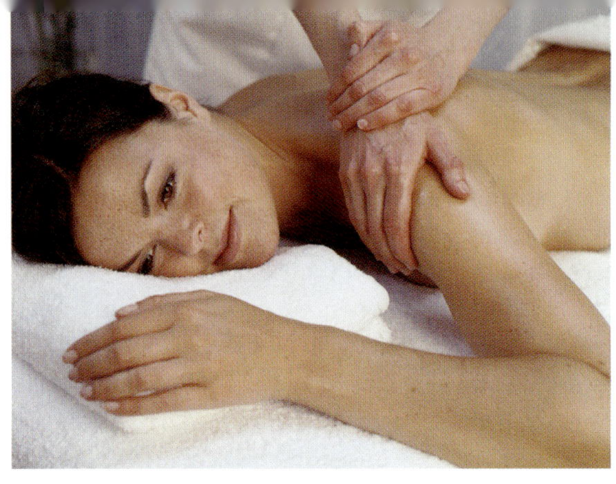

affect us through smell.

Research has established that some chemical constituents of essential oils are absorbed by inhalation, while further studies also suggest that absorption through the skin can occur when inhalation is prevented. However there is no proof that all, or any, constituents of essential oils will travel to a given organ and cause a specific effect.

ARE THEY SAFE TO USE?

There is a common misconception that 'natural' means 'safe'. Essential oils are highly concentrated, and, while most represent little or no risk when correctly used, some constituents can be toxic in large quantities, or can adversely affect people with particular conditions.

An understanding of the chemistry of essential oils is of vital importance to professional aromatherapists. In addition, the aromatherapist should always take a thorough medical history during consultation with a client so that a safe combination of oils is used.

The risks associated with certain oils – and the fact that the quantities in which most essential oils are sold (5-15ml) can be lethal if drunk by a young child – also make it important that anyone using oils at home does so with caution (read more about this in Chapter Six).

There is much debate about what is, and what is not, safe when it comes to using essential oils. The list opposite errs on the side of caution. However, it is probably the best advice for anyone new to aromatherapy to follow.

You should consult a qualified aromatherapist and your doctor before using essential oils if you are pregnant, if you have epilepsy or a heart condition, if you are asthmatic, if you suffer from a skin condition, allergy or generally sensitive skin, and if you are taking conventional medication or a homoeopathic remedy.

Infants and young children have delicate skin, so only extremely well-diluted oils should be used.

Citrus oils increase our skin's sensitivity to the sun, so you should avoid exposure to the sun (or a sunbed) for at least six hours after using these.

Essential oils with relaxing properties can cause drowsiness. Therefore, they should not be used if you are going to drive or if you intend to use machinery shortly afterwards.

AROMATHERAPY CAUTION!

Essential oils that should never be used at home because they are potentially very toxic include:

- Arnica
- Bitter almond
- Boldo leaf
- Broom
- Buchu
- Calamus
- Camphor (brown, yellow, and white)
- Chervil
- Cinnamon bark
- Horseradish
- Jaborandi
- Mountain (dwarf) pine
- Mugwort
- Narcissus
- Pennyroyal
- Rue
- Sassafras
- Savine
- Tansy
- Thuja
- Tonka
- Wintergreen
- Wormseed
- Wormwood

Some of these may be used in perfumes, food flavourings and medicines, and, even on occasion, by experienced aromatherapists; and the plants they are extracted from may well be used in cooking, herbal or homoeopathic medicines.

AROMATHERAPY OILS

There are about 200 essential oils produced commercially, of which some 50-100 are used in aromatherapy. Some of the more commonly used essential oils are described below.

BERGAMOT
Citrus bergamia
Aroma: Citrus, fresh, lively.
Properties: Refreshing, relaxing, anti-septic, anti-depressant.
Used for: Anxiety, mild depression, improving moods, grief, loss of appetite, urinary problems, acne, oily skin.
Cautions: Photosensitisation and skin irritation.

CAMOMILE, BLUE (GERMAN)
Matricaria recutia
Aroma: Fruity, herbaceous, pungent.
Properties: Anti-inflammatory, anti-bacterial, anti-spasmodic, calming.
Used for: Bronchitis, lung problems, hay fever, allergies, skin problems, wounds, muscle stiffness, joint pain, nervous tension, stress, menstrual problems, digestion.

Cautions: Avoid during pregnancy; mild skin irritation.

CAMOMILE, ROMAN
Chamaemelum nobile
Aroma: Fruity, herbaceous.
Properties: Anti-inflammatory, anti-bacterial, calming, relaxing, sedative.
Used for: As for blue camomile, insomnia, tension headaches.
Cautions: As for blue camomile.

CLARY SAGE
Salvia sclarea
Aroma: Musky, warm, hay-like, herbaceous.
Properties: Anti-septic, astringent, anti-depressant, relaxing, sedative.
Used for: Depression, anxiety, stress, depression, panic, shock, skin disorders, menstrual and menopausal problems, muscular tension.
Cautions: Avoid during pregnancy; drowsiness.

EUCALYPTUS
Eucalyptus globules
Aroma: Camphor-like, sweet, woody, powerful.

Properties: Anti-septic, anti-spasmodic, stimulating, uplifting.

Used for: Respiratory tract problems, nasal congestion, chest infections, colds, flu, muscular aches, joint pain, urinary tract infections, mood uplifting, lethargy, insect repellent.

Cautions: Avoid in early pregnancy; toxic if consumed; avoid in massage.

GERANIUM

Pelargonium graveolens
Aroma: Floral, sweet.

Properties: Anti-septic, astringent, tonic, circulatory, balancing (can stimulate or relax), anti-depressant.

Used for: Relaxation, mood uplifting, for confidence and self-esteem, nervous tension, skin problems, herpes, menstrual and menopausal problems, balancing hormones.

Cautions: Skin irritation.

LAVENDER

Lavandula angustifolia or L. officinalis
Aroma: Floral, herbaceous, sweet.

Properties: Anti-septic, anti-spasmodic, anti-depressant, pain-relieving, anti-nausea, relaxing, sedative.

Used for: As one of the most versatile oils, there is little it cannot be used for, but it is particularly helpful for relaxation, headaches, burns, colds, catarrh, skin problems, menstrual problems.

Cautions: Avoid in early pregnancy; mild skin irritation.

MARJORAM, SWEET
Origanum majorana
Aroma: Camphor-like, warm, sweet.

Properties: Anti-bacterial, anti-spasmodic, pain-relieving, calming, sedative.

Used for: Muscular problems, arthritis, rheumatism, headaches, migraine, insomnia, anxiety, grief, depression, digestive problems, nasal and sinus congestion.

Cautions: Avoid during pregnancy.

PATCHOULI
Pogostemon cablin
Aroma: Musky, sweet, woody, balsamic.

Properties: Anti-septic, anti-bacterial, anti-viral, anti-depressant, anti-inflammatory, astringent, stimulating, uplifting, stomach calming, aphrodisiac.
Used for: Stress, depression, lethargy, skin care and problems, oily hair, scalp problems, fungal infections.
Cautions: Possible headaches.

PEPPERMINT
Mentha piperita
Aroma: Menthol-like, powerful.
Properties: Anti-septic, anti-spasmodic, pain-relieving, nerve tonic, digestive, stimulating, uplifting.
Used for: Clearing the mind, concentration, bruises, itchy skin conditions, indigestion, flatulence, nausea, diarrhoea, period pains, headaches.
Cautions: Avoid in early pregnancy.

ROSE
Rosa damascena, R. centifolia
Aroma: Rosy, floral, intense.
Properties: Anti-septic, anti-depressant, anti-spasmodic, nerve tonic, relaxing, sedative.

Used for: Mild depression, nervous palpitations, negative emotions, fears, anxiety, skin care, skin problems, headaches, insomnia, menstrual problems, hangovers.
Cautions: Avoid during pregnancy.

ROSEMARY
Rosmarinus officinalis
Aroma: Fresh, herbaceous.
Properties: Anti-septic, anti-spasmodic, astringent, tonic, pain-relieving, tissue-warming, stimulating, refreshing.
Used for: Muscular stiffness and aches, arthritis, neuralgia, poor circulation, headaches, gout, water retention, skin problems, mental fatigue, poor memory.

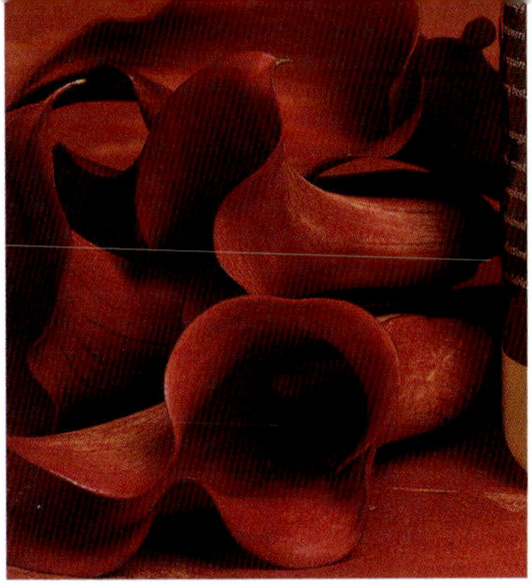

Rose essential oil can be used to treat mild depression and anxiety.

Cautions: Avoid during pregnancy and if you have epilepsy or high blood pressure.

SANDALWOOD
Santalum album

Aroma: Woody, balsamic, sweet.

Properties: Anti-septic, anti-depressant, anti-microbial, astringent, tonic, aphrodisiac, relaxing, sedative.

Used for: Worry, fear, negative emotions, stress, skin problems, throat and chest infections, urinary infections.

Cautions: None.

TEA TREE
Melaleuca alternifolia

Aroma: Medicinal, fresh, spicy.

Properties: Anti-septic, anti-bacterial, anti-viral, anti-fungal, deodorant, stimulating.

Used for: Infectious conditions, cuts, sores, herpes, ulcers, bites, skin problems, haemorrhoids, minor burns, thrush, candida, fungal vaginitis, muscular pain, athlete's foot, colds, flu, dandruff, halitosis, shock, panic, mind stimulant.

Cautions: Mild skin irritant; can cause dizziness with deep inhalation.

THYME
Thymus vulgaris
Aroma: Herby, fresh.
Properties: Anti-septic, anti-microbial, stimulating.
Used for: Colds, flu, bronchial infections, sore throats, strengthening the immune system, circulatory problems, rheumatic aches and pains, mental and physical fatigue, depression, insomnia.
Cautions: Avoid during pregnancy; skin irritation.

YLANG YLANG
Cananga odorata
Aroma: Jasmine-like, floral, smoky.
Properties: Anti-septic, anti-fungal, anti-depressant, hypotensive (reduces blood pressure), relaxing, calming, deodorant, aphrodisiac.
Used for: Stress, mild depression, negative emotions, stress, stress-related high blood pressure, hyperventilation, anxiety, hyperactivity, skin care and skin problems.
Cautions: Avoid in early pregnancy; can cause headaches and nausea.

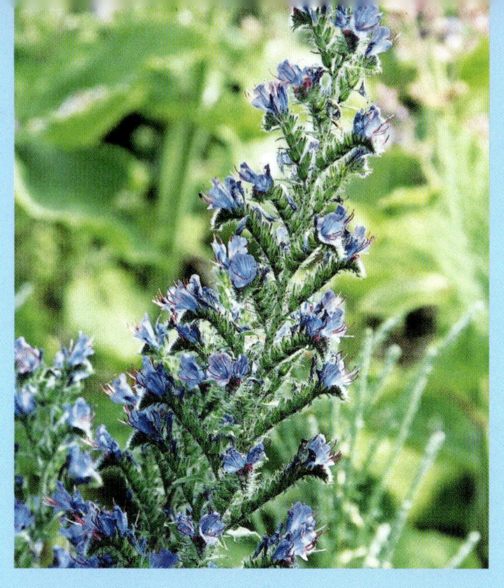

4 Will Aromatherapy Work For Me?

Aromatherapy claims success in treating a wide range of health problems.

Below are some case studies, which may help you to decide if aromatherapy can be of help to you.

STRESS AND TENSION HEADACHES

Aromatherapy is said to be particularly helpful for stress and stress-related problems, such as insomnia, restlessness, anxiety, mild depression, headaches and migraine.

Angela is 27, single, and newly promoted to a head of department in her company. While the promotion was hard earned, Angela was finding the extra responsibility and workload increasingly stressful. By the end of each day, she was suffering from tension headaches. At night she had trouble relaxing, and sleep often seemed impossible.

Angela sought help from an aromatherapist, who gave her

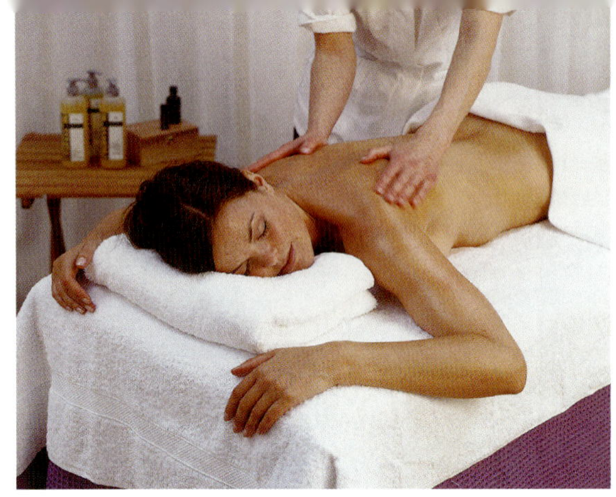

Aromatherapy massages are a great way of easing stress and tension.

a massage using a blend of geranium, lavender, sandalwood and ylang ylang. She suggested that Angela used the same blend in a vaporizer in-between treatments, to help release tension and to encourage sound sleep.

She encouraged Angela to look at her diet and recommended that she took regular exercise – perhaps by getting off the bus a few stops earlier, or by using stairs rather than lifts. She also recommended that Angela discussed her workload and training with her supervisor.

Angela returned for two further treatments, after which she reported that she felt much more in control of her life and generally more relaxed and healthy.

RESPIRATORY PROBLEMS

Asthma and other respiratory conditions (such as the common cold and influenza) are all said to respond well to treatment with aromatherapy.

Chris has two children: Ben aged seven and Orla aged five. Both are prone to colds in the winter. Chris finds that essential oils are helpful in treating the symptoms, as both children like 'the smelling medicine'.

If one child does get a cold, despite the preventive steps Chris takes (such as ensuring a regular intake of foods rich in vitamin C) she adds one drop each of peppermint, eucalyptus and tea tree to a bowl of hot water and gets the child to inhale under a towel every evening. Chris also finds that, during the day, a drop of lemon oil on a tissue helps to clear the head.

WOMEN'S HEALTH

Many women's health problems can be readily improved with aromatherapy. These include menstrual problems, thrush, and menopausal problems. There are also oils that can be helpful during pregnancy, labour and postnatally.

Gloria had always received regular aromatherapy, and, when she became pregnant with her first child, she was keen to continue with regular treatments. Her therapist agreed to work with her, and her midwife was also supportive.

Over her pregnancy Gloria received regular massages, which were gradually adapted to take in her changing shape and the positions she could comfortably lie and sit in. Her aromatherapist also made suggestions for oils that could help with Gloria's nausea in the first few months. Gloria experimented with emotionally balancing oils, such as geranium and mandarin, in her essence burner to help her cope with the emotional changes she was experiencing. During labour Gloria's partner, Moses,

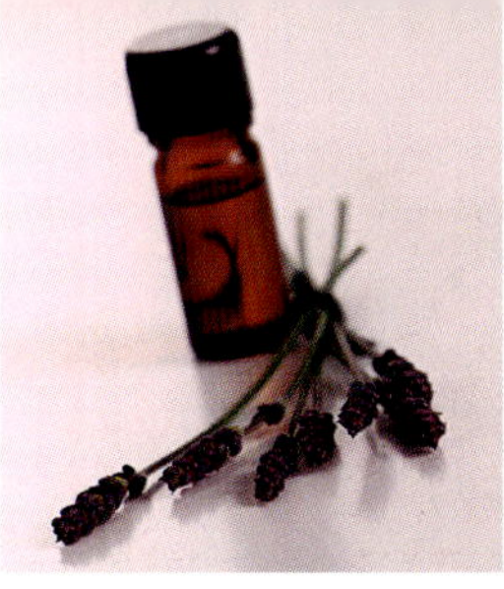

Lavender oil in the bath is very soothing.

regularly massaged her back and tummy with a blend of camomile, mandarin and sandalwood, which Gloria reported was very helpful. Postnatally, Gloria added a blend of cypress and lavender to her baths to ease the bruising she developed from the birth of her son, Eden.

SKIN CONDITIONS

Burns, eczema, psoriasis and many other skin conditions can be relieved by the use of essential oils. Wound and scar healing can also be improved with aromatherapy.

Brian had suffered from acne since he was a teenager. When his girlfriend suggested that he try aromatherapy, he was open to a new approach.

Over a period of six months Brian had regular treatments with the aromatherapist. He also agreed to some helpful dietary changes, including a reduction in spicy and fatty food – especially dairy products. He also increased the amount of water he drank.

Between treatments, the aromatherapist made up a blend of juniper berry and atlas cedarwood that Brian could add to spring water to bathe his skin. He was also given a blend of lemon, petitgrain and atlas cedarwood to add to jojoba carrier oil to use as a soothing lotion.

Brian's acne responded well to the new regime. He decided to continue with regular appointments because they made him much more relaxed as well as keeping his spots under control.

ARTHRITIS

Aromatherapists have also claimed success in the treatment of conditions such as arthritis, muscular and neuralgic pain, digestive disorders and constipation.

Arthur, in his early sixties, had suffered arthritic pain in his shoulders for some years. He had felt it was an inevitable part of growing older and that there was little that could be done for him. However, a new GP at Arthur's surgery suggested that he see an aromatherapist.

With nothing to lose, Arthur made an appointment with a therapist recommended by the GP. He had treatments

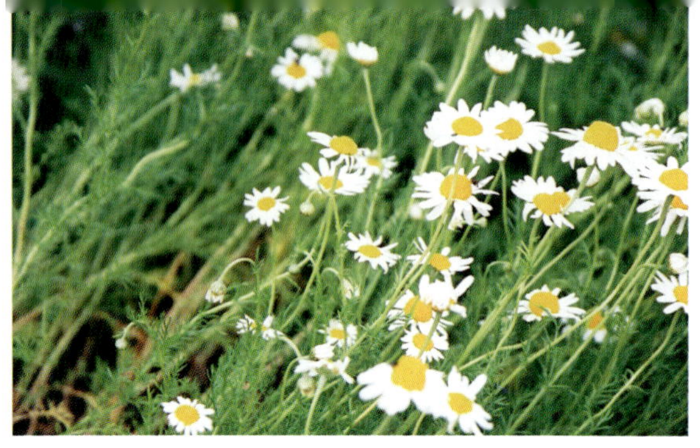

Camomile, blended with other essential oils, can help to relieve the pain of arthritis.

regularly for three months, after which he reported to his GP that he was completely pain-free.

The aromatherapist had used a blend of oils, including lavender and rosemary, and had recommended that Arthur used a blend of lavender, rosemary, eucalyptus and camomile in his bath at night, if the pain was particularly bad between treatments.

Arthur has continued to see the aromatherapist regularly to make sure that the pain does not return.

FIRST-AID ESSENTIAL OILS

Several essential oils deserve a place in everyone's medical cupboard. While not a comprehensive list, my own favourites include:

LAVENDER

This is good for:

- **Minor burns:** always immerse burns in cold water until the pain subsides, but then try applying a small amount of neat lavender to gain extra relief and to avoid unnecessary scarring.
- **Bruises, cuts and grazes:** wounds should be cleaned with fresh, cool water, but a cold compress with lavender is very soothing afterwards.
- **Jetlag and insomnia:** a drop of lavender oil on your pillow or a tissue will help to promote sleep.
- **Headaches:** try massaging a few drops of lavender oil into your temples to relieve headaches.

TEA TREE

Try tea tree for:
- **Chilblains:** apply a drop of neat tea tree to the affected area, or massage the foot with a combination of 10ml grapeseed oil and five drops of tea tree.
- **Cold sores:** dilute the tea tree in a carrier oil and dab it on the affected areas with a cotton wool bud.
- **Earache:** dilute the oil in a carrier oil and massage around your ear and jaw (try also lavender and Roman camomile).
- **Bruises, cuts and grazes:** use as an alternative to lavender.
- **Insect bites and stings:** apply one drop of tea tree (or lavender) to the affected area after pulling out the sting with tweezers (if visible).

PEPPERMINT

Use peppermint for:
- **Flagging concentration:** try either a drop on a tissue to sniff, or add peppermint to an essence burner for an instant pick-me-up.

HOMEMADE TOILETRIES

BATH OILS

For one full bath, mix six drops of essential oil(s) with 5ml of a carrier oil (sweet almond, grapeseed or hazelnut). For a relaxing evening bath, try a mixture of four drops lavender and two drops marjoram, or four drops camomile and two drops lavender. If you feel particularly tired in the morning, try a pick-me-up bath with two drops of thyme, three drops of rosemary and one drop of peppermint.

SKIN CREAM

Melt 20g of almond carrier oil and 10g shredded beeswax in a pyrex bowl over a pan of gently heating water. Remove from heat and add 40g of rosewater or distilled water very slowly, beating the mixture continuously. When the water has been absorbed, transfer the mixture to a clean glass jar and add your own essential oils. Oils suitable for most skins include rose, geranium and lavender.

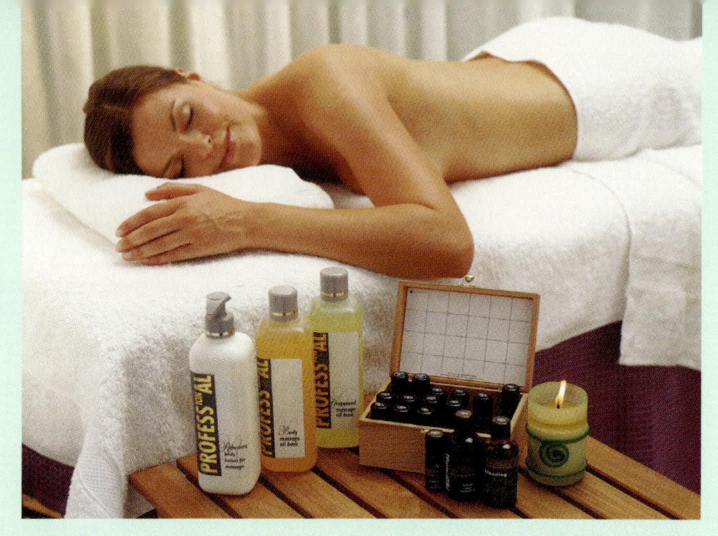

5 Going To An Aromatherapist

Where do you find a qualified therapist?

Personal recommendation is the best option, but there are also organisations and associations that can provide you with the names and addresses of local aromatherapists (see page 60).

WHAT TO EXPECT

Before your appointment it is a good idea to have bathed, although you should avoid highly scented bath products. You should also avoid a large meal and alcohol immediately prior to the appointment.

The first time you visit an aromatherapist you will be asked for some personal details (e.g. name, age and occupation), details about your health problem (how long you have had it? When and how it affects you) and details of any previous or current treatment, etc. Your aromatherapist will also want to know about your previous medical history, including any serious illnesses, accidents or operations, and any allergies or other minor complaints. In addition, you may be asked about your lifestyle (e.g. diet, exercise, smoking and drinking habits, and your current stress levels).

These questions are asked because it is important for the aromatherapist to establish that there are no reasons why you should not receive treatment.

THE THERAPIST

Aromatherapists are not trained in clinical diagnosis. They work from the diagnosis you have already received from your doctor and the additional information you have given them.

Some therapists are trained in other complementary therapies, such as reflexology or iridology, which will allow them to identify areas of weakness in your body that would respond to treatment.

Some aromatherapists use dowsing, which involves using the swing of a pendulum to indicate the most appropriate oils. Other therapists rely on intuition and experience. A technique called muscle-testing, which helps to indicate which of the major organs are weak and which oils would help most, may also be used.

CHOOSING THE OILS

After the consultation, your aromatherapist will mix your individual blend of essential oils in a vegetable oil base (a 'carrier' oil), which will be designed to work on a physical, mental, emotional and even spiritual level at the same time. This blend will usually be used in a full-body massage during your treatment, but you may also be advised to use it in baths and inhalations at home.

You may be asked which oil or oils you prefer out of a small selection, as individual preferences vary and it is important that you like the aroma of the oils selected.

AROMATHERAPY MASSAGE

What part of your body is massaged depends on your problem. In most cases a whole-body massage will be offered, which will take about an hour. However, someone who is very ill may only have their hands or feet massaged.

Some therapists will give the massage on a treatment couch, whereas others prefer to work on the floor. All should ensure that the treatment room (and their hands) are warm, as clients will usually undress to some degree. It is important that you feel relaxed, and a therapist should ensure your body is not unnecessarily exposed.

NUMBER OF TREATMENTS

How many treatments you will need is something your therapist will discuss with you.

POST TREATMENT

After your treatment you may feel a little disorientated or light-headed; you may feel more energetic or relaxed. Schedule your appointment so that you have few, if any, commitments afterwards.

Some people find that they have a short reaction period when they actually feel worse – usually within 24 hours. If this happens to you, you should feel better within two days of your treatment. You should then go on to experience a steady improvement in your problem – and general health – from week to week.

You should not bathe or use sunbeds for at least six hours after treatment, because some oils make the skin more sensitive to the sun.

HOLISTIC HEALTH CARE

Most aromatherapists will emphasise the importance of taking a holistic approach to health. By this, they mean that, for essential oils to exercise their revitalising and balancing powers to the full, your body and mind must be in a receptive state. Poor diet, too much alcohol, a smoking habit and lack of exercise can all cause toxins to accumulate in your body. Add high levels of stress and muscular tension and you have a recipe for ill health. While aromatherapy will help alleviate such symptoms, for long-term benefits essential oils need to be combined with a balanced lifestyle that should include a nutritious diet and regular exercise.

6

Using Essential Oils At Home

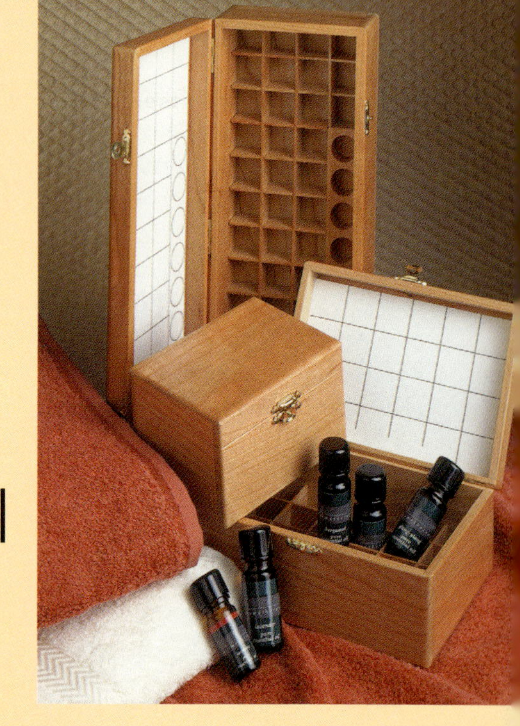

Although most essential oils are safe for home use, there are some basic safety guidelines that everyone should follow.

Essential oils should:

- Be kept out of reach of children and pets.
- Be stored away from naked flames (they are flammable).
- Never be taken internally.
- Always be diluted in a carrier oil before use, unless otherwise stated.

Spilt, undiluted essential oils should be washed off the skin with washing-up liquid, and from eyes with warm water. To avoid skin irritation or an allergic reaction, a patch test is recommended before using an oil for the first time. Place a drop of diluted essential oil on the inside of your wrist or elbow, and cover with a plaster for 12 hours. If, after this time, there is any redness or itching, the oil should not be used. An adverse reaction can be eased with a little almond oil, which can be washed off later. If the reaction persists, a visit to the doctor may be necessary.

BUYING AND STORING OILS

Aromatherapists recommend using only pure essential oils. Some products may be labelled as 'aromatherapy oils'. but these often have only a small percentage of essential oil included and they do not always represent good value for money.

To make sure you have a pure oil, check the label, and, if you are still not sure, try smelling it. If it stings your nostrils, it is likely to be synthetic.

Qualified therapists can also recommend particular brands if you feel confused about the products available.

Essential oils must be stored properly in order to retain their therapeutic properties. They should be kept in dark glass bottles in a cool, dark place. The bottle tops should be tightly closed to prevent the oils evaporating.

As most oils deteriorate after approximately two years, aromatherapists recommend adding the date of purchase to the label after buying an oil.

BLENDING

Essential oils are usually diluted in base or carrier oils. Cold-pressed vegetable oils are best because no solvents or heat have been used in the extraction process. For home use, lighter vegetable oils are good all-purpose carriers.

Inexpensive light oils include sunflower, safflower, corn and soya. Equally versatile, but more expensive, light oils include almond, grapeseed, apricot kernel, coconut and hazelnut.

Blends of carrier oil and essential oils are usually divided into normal ($2\frac{1}{2}$ per cent) and low (1 per cent) dilutions. For a normal dilution, 10 drops of essential oil are added to 20ml of carrier oil (enough for a full body massage). For babies and children, it is recommended that you seek professional help.

Blends should be stored in dark glass bottles that can be tightly sealed. If kept in the fridge, they will last for several months. The blend should always be shaken well before use.

USING OILS

Most home remedies for common ailments will specify the most beneficial way of using the essential oil. Massage is the most common use. For home use it is important that the person offering the massage has received some training in the techniques involved.

Skin lotions and oils can be added to a simple cold cream or to a richer carrier oil. The mixture should be applied with a gentle circular motion.

Adding oils to a bath is by far the easiest route for home use.

Up to six drops of essential oil, or mix of oils, can be added to a warm bath (if the water is too hot, the oils will quickly evaporate). The essential oil should be thoroughly dispersed in the water before you relax in the bath for up to 20 minutes. People with sensitive skin can dilute the oils in a carrier oil before adding to their bath.

Vaporisation is an easy and effective way of dispersing essential oils throughout your home – to freshen the air or to create a particular ambiance. Three to six drops of essential oil can be dropped into a bowl of hot water or a specially designed essence burner. Or up to 10 drops of essential oil can be added to a plant spray filled with fresh spring water, but avoid polished surfaces, as the oils may stain.

To inhale the aromas, add up to six drops of essential oil to a bowl of hot water and inhale the steam under a towel.

One drop of essential oil can be safely applied to a pillow (e.g. lavender to help sleep), clothing or a tissue, although it is worth testing on a hem first to ensure there is no staining.

Aromatherapists do not recommend applying undiluted oils to the skin, with the honorable exceptions of lavender oil for burns, insect bites and cuts, tea tree oil for spots and fungal infections, and lemon oil for warts and verrucas.

Six drops of essential oil can be added to a bowl of hot or ice-cold water to create a compress. Soak a clean cotton cloth in the solution, squeeze out the excess water, and apply to the affected area.

Further Information

The following bodies will be able to help you find an aromatherapist in your area and provide you with more information about aromatherapy.

AROMATHERAPY AND
ALLIED PRACTITIONERS'
ASSOCIATION
8 George Street,
Croydon, Surrey, CR0 1PA.
Tel: 020 8680 7761

Web: www.aromatherapyuk.net
Email:
aromatherapyuk@aol.com

ASSOCIATION OF MEDICAL
AROMATHERAPISTS
11 Park Circus,
Glasgow, G3 6AX.
Tel: 0141 3324924
Web: www.complementary
medicinecentre.co.uk
Email: complementarymedicine
centre@compuserve.com

AROMATHERAPY COUNCIL
PO Box 19834,
London, SE25 6WF.
Tel. 0208 251 7912
Web: www.aromatherapy-
regulation.org.uk/
Email: info@aromatherapy-
regulation.org.uk

INTERNATIONAL
FEDERATION OF
PROFESSIONAL
AROMATHERAPISTS
IFPA House,

82 Ashby Road, Hinckley,
Leics, LE10 1SN.
Tel: 01455 637987
Web: www.ifparoma.org
Email: admin@ifparoma.org

INTERNATIONAL
FEDERATION OF
AROMATHERAPISTS
182 Chiswick High Road,
London, W4 1PP.
Tel. 020 8742 2605
Web: www.ifaroma.co.uk
Email: office@ifaroma.org

About the author

Joanna Trevelyan is an experienced journalist with a particular interest in complementary therapies, health and nursing, environmental health issues, and women's issues. She has written for a wide range of professional bodies, including the World Health Organisation, the Natural Medicines Society, the Parliamentary Group for Complementary and Alternative Medicine, and the Foundation for Integrated Health.

Joanna has also been the editor of the professional journal *Nursing Times*. In 1994, she was awarded a Commendation in the Medical Journalism Awards.

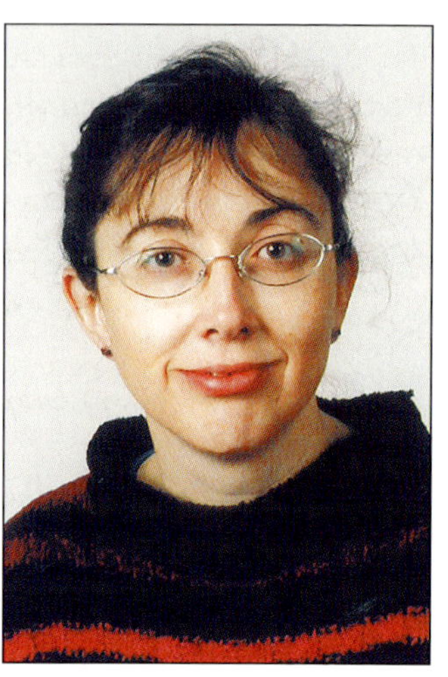

ACKNOWLEDGEMENTS
Photography courtesy of Dick Smith, with special thanks due to Tisserand Aromatherapy Products Limited for further help with photographs.

Other titles in the series

- **Understanding Acupressure**
- **Understanding Acupuncture**
- **Understanding The Alexander Technique**
- **Understanding Aloe Vera**
- **Understanding Bach Flower Remedies**
- **Understanding The Bowen Technique**
- **Understanding Craniosacral Therapy**
- **Understanding Echinacea**
- **Understanding Evening Primrose**
- **Understanding Fish Oils**
- **Understanding Garlic**
- **Understanding Ginseng**
- **Understanding Head Massage**
- **Understanding Kinesiology**
- **Understanding Lavender**
- **Understanding Massage**
- **Understanding Pilates**
- **Understanding Reflexology**
- **Understanding Reiki**
- **Understanding St. John's Wort**
- **Understanding Shiatsu**
- **Understanding Yoga**

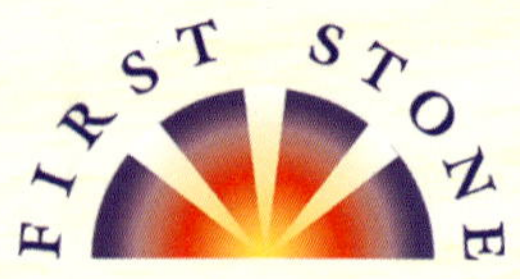

First published 2005 by First Stone Publishing
PO Box 8, Lydney, Gloucestershire, GL15 6YD

The contents of this book are for information only and are not intended as a substitute for appropriate medical attention. The author and publishers admit no liability for any consequences arising from following any advice contained within this book. If you have any concerns about your health or medication, always consult your doctor.

ISBN 1 904439 17 9

Printed and bound in Hong Kong through Printworks International Ltd.